Karen's
Health, Nutrition,
&
Fitness Manual

By Karen Minnis

DEDICATION

To God be the glory for the things he has done.

CONTENTS

Karen's Health, Nutrition, & Fitness Manual

ABOUT THE AUTHOR

Karen Minnis is an aerobics instructor certified by *A/R Christian Aerobics* having completed their *Jump Start Program* July 10, 2001

To hear her aerobics routine music CDs go to:

http://www.cdbaby.com/wtlclub6

&

http://www.cdbaby.com/wtlclub4

The Music is performed by *The WTL Club*
(The Way, Truth & Life Club. The band is comprised of Karen, her husband and children.) To hear more of their music, go to:
http://www.cdbaby.com/all/thewtlclub

Also, Karen Minnis completed the Professional Career Development Institute's *"Professional Fitness and Nutrition Program"* and received her diploma on April 22, 1997 from their *School of Fitness & Nutrition.*

Karen's Health, Nutrition, & Fitness Manual is a composite of various articles Karen has written and her teachings are biblically based from a Christian perspective using a common sense approach to healthy living.

Karen Minnis and her husband Michael were married in 1983; she is the mother of four children, Michael, Christy, Joshua & Melissa; they are all grow-ups. They help out in the gardens, farmer's market and food pantry and so do some of the grand-children.

ACKNOWLEDGMENTS

Karen Minnis is the Executive Director of Landmark Training Development Company ("Landmark").
http://landmarktraining.webs.com Landmark operates several entities, including an urban farming facility in the Orange Mound community of Memphis, Tennessee which is comprised of Landmark Food Pantry that has been open 5 days per week since 2011 providing emergency food to those in need. Landmark Gardens is an organic based training farm that produces over two tons of food annually and includes 3 high-tunnels, a chicken coop, several fruit trees and a beekeeping operation.

Landmark Farmers Market is a licensed food manufacturer located adjacent to the food pantry and gardens. It is open year round offering natural remedies and herbal teas whose ingredients are grown on-site. Landmark Skin Cream and Lip Balm are proprietary products that are manufactured on-site as well as chow-chow and salsa.   Karen is a certified food processor and offers food canning classes several times per year.
Go to: http://www.landmarkfarmersmarket.com

1 CHAPTER

<u>NUTRITION BASICS</u>

Today our diets are full of processed foods; foods that man has tampered with, not to benefit our bodies, but to give the food a longer shelf life to increase corporate profits. We are eating fast foods which are filled with fat, salt, sugar and consequently, we are eating ourselves to death. High combinations of processed foods is a primary cause of obesity and contribute to heart disease, high blood pressure, diabetes and cancer. One of the most commonly used food processing agents is partially hydrogenated oil (fat). Foods we do not need to prepare, just heat and eat, are typically filled with partially hydrogenated oil (fat).

Partially hydrogenated fat comes from oil that would normally be liquid at room temperature but has been chemically processed to become solid at room temperature. Thus, creating a longer shelf life in food. Partially hydrogenated fat poses a greater threat for clogging our blood & arteries than butter, lard and other saturated fats that are naturally solid at room temperature. So, you may ask, what is a reasonable solution to not eating microwave meals? Get back to the basics! Eating fresh fruits, vegetables, whole foods and drinking plenty of water is an excellent basic nutritional plan.

Also, we need to consider that most whole foods which are not organically grown do not have as much health and vitality in them as they would if farm land were given a chance to rest every 7th year. God said in Leviticus, chapter 25, verses 3 thru 6 that we should work the land 6 years and let the land rest the 7th year. However, God has allowed man to use technology to put herbs, vitamins and minerals in concentrated liquid or pill form so that we may use such supplements to provide balance in our nutritional needs. We should supplement our diets with the advice of qualified health professionals.

I encourage you to read food product labels and educate yourself on good nutritional values. You only get one body and it makes good sense to take care of it. The closer a food product is to its natural state, the higher its quality... the higher quality food can help maintain health as well as quicken recovery from sickness. Eat fresh and natural foods because in this state, all of the enzymes are found intact. The amino acids are in their finest form, the minerals, vitamins, trace elements or "life force" are all present and in turn, are capable of helping you to maintain and/or reproduce healthy tissue.

2 CHAPTER

A GOOD DIETARY FOUNDATION

Are you drinking enough water? Our bodily composition is over 70% water. Water is needed and used for every cell, tissue and organ of our bodies. It is essential that we provide sufficient amounts of water for our bodily needs. Plus, the regular consumption of fruits and vegetables provide an abundance of nutrients for every cell of our bodies. If we are not consuming sufficient amounts of water, fruits and vegetables, we are lacking in a good dietary foundation.

In the wilderness, God gave the children of Israel exactly what they needed to survive. The children of Israel wanted more than what God had already given them for the moment. Although God had given them exactly what they needed to survive. (See "Psalms 78:23-31")

God has given us everything that we need but we don't want water, fruits and vegetables, we want fast foods, donuts, soda pop, etc. We complain that fruits and veggies aren't exciting enough. We want something different than what he's given us. Are we like the children of Israel? We want what we want and not what we need, or do we want what's best for us. Let us wake up and find and follow Jesus - the Way, the Truth, & the Life. (See "John 14:6")

3 CHAPTER

THE ORIGINAL FAST FOOD DIET

'Fast foods' are not just a 21th century thing. They have been around since before man was created. The original 'fast food' diet was fresh raw herbs, fruits and vegetables, nuts & grains. What's faster than peeling a banana and eating it, or eating some grapes, or strawberries or an apple.

We have no excuse for not eating right, because God made it easy for us from the beginning. The Bible says in Genesis 1:29 "And God said, "See, I have given you every herb that yields seed which is on the face of all the earth, and every tree whose fruit yields seed; to you it shall be for food."

Fresh raw fruits and vegetables have live enzymes in them which help to heal, cleanse, & revitalize us. The live enzymes that are in the raw foods that we should consume every day are like soap to our insides. A day without some fresh raw foods is like a day without a bath or shower - if we go too many days everyone will know.

We need, along with all of the other things that we consume every day, at least 5 to 9 servings of fresh raw fruits and vegetables every day; not to mention the 6 to 8 glasses of water that we need every day (which we'll talk about in more detail later). Have you had yours today? Plan ahead and be prepared whether you go to school, work, or even the doctor's office. Bon appetite!

4 CHAPTER

<u>LIVE TO EAT OR EAT TO LIVE</u>

I would like to give you something to sink your teeth into - late night eating. Late night eating can make a difference of 5 to 10 lbs in a year. Add that 5 to 10 lbs. a year for a few years and it could be the reason that you weigh what you weigh.

There are a lot of people that have a habit of eating late night meals and thinking nothing of it. There are some that are trying to lose weight, who get a good workout in and then feel justified in eating a late night meal because they think that they've earned it by working out - or just because they haven't eaten dinner - whether they're hungry or not.

Our food needs at least 2 hours of digestion time before we go to sleep (3 or 4 would be ideal - especially if we've eaten meat). Digestion takes a lot of work for our bodies - which is why, after we eat an especially large meal, all that we want to do is nap.

If we cut back on late night eating and start eating breakfast, we would be more energetic in the morning. (Most late night eaters have a hard time getting up in the mornings because their bodies had to work so hard while they were sleeping.). This one simple change could make the difference of 5-10 lbs. a year. If you do need a late night snack, have some fruit. Watery fruits like orange & apples are in and out of your stomachs in 20 minutes. Heavier fruits like bananas & raisins in 40 minutes.

Another idea is to eat fruit alone and only on an empty stomach because it is in & out of your stomach in such a short period of time. Other foods could take 2 - 4 hours to digest. Meats take the longest to digest.

Karen Minnis

Sometimes fruits are blamed for gas and indigestion. The problem probably is that you've mixed the fruit with some other foods which has caused it to rot in your stomach.

Fruit is the easiest food to digest in your body because of the enzymes & its basic chemical make-up.

Think about slowing down when you eat. We rush to eat meals sometimes, even when we don't have to because it has become a habit. If we slow down to eat, it will be easier on our bodies as far as digestion, because the more we chew & break down our food into tiny pieces, the less work our body has to do in the form of digestion. Just imagine - all digestion takes place with digestive juices, therefore everything that we eat has to be broken down with these juices. If we want to lose weight, we need to definitely chew our foods better, because we will require less food to be satisfied & over time it will translate into lbs. off in the long run.

Last but not least; Realize that you are body, soul, & spirit. A lot of our bodies are overweight, but our spirits are mal-nourished - even anorexic because we make sure that our bodies get 3 square meals, but we virtually starve our spirits. We might give our spirits a snack on Sunday by going to church.

Think about it - is God first in your life? Are you giving Him His just desserts? Jesus is The Way, The Truth, and The Life. Your quality of life will be so much better when you make Him Lord of your life.

5 CHAPTER

PLAN TO EAT RIGHT

So many people complain that they don't have the time, the money, &/or the know-how to eat right. We all have everything that we need - we just have to do it. When we don't plan ahead, we plan to fail.

First of all, when it comes to the time to eat right, the only way that it is going to happen is that we plan ahead. If you are always rushed in the mornings & don't have time to fix breakfast, snacks, &/or lunch for the day, prepare ahead the night before. When you plan ahead, you won't be caught without & have to eat whatever you can find or run out to get food which will probably be more costly & less nutritious than what you could have brought from home.

Take your breakfast with you if necessary. Fruit is fantastic for breakfast, lunch &/or snacks (eat 1 or more pieces in a sitting). Toast, bagels, yogurt, oatmeal, and whole grain/fiber cereals, are all wonderful for breakfast. You can prepare protein smoothies by freezing bananas without the peel & adding them with other fruits &/or juices &/or whey or vegetable protein powders to make a filling breakfast drink.

For lunch, you can pack nutritious left-overs from dinner, prepare salad ingredients ahead and put them together the night before. Prepare a large pot of hearty vegetable soup & freeze it in one-serving size bowls for a quick lunch, snack or dinner meal. Nut butter & jelly sandwiches are great.

Snacks can be fruit, carrot & celery sticks, boiled eggs, granola bars, protein bars, yogurt, dates, prunes, & raisins. When it comes to money, buy fruits & vegetables only when they are on sale. Some larger super stores honor the sales of other stores for one-stop shopping.

For dinner, you can slow cook some meals (beans, stews, soups, roasts) at night & they will be ready before work the next morning. You can cook enough for 2 or 3 meals at one time so that you don't have to cook every day & can keep a variety of things in the freezer for quick heat up.

Know-how is just a matter of eating only the things that you know are good for you and following the rules of keeping it simple, sweetie. 50-70% of our diets should be fresh, raw fruits & veggies. Get back to the basics. We need 5 - 9 servings of fruits & veggies every day. When we get all of our servings of them on a regular basis we will feel much better & save time, money, & our health.

6 CHAPTER

NO MORE CRASH DIETING

The big buzz right now is to lose weight fast & lose weight now! It is vital that we learn the proper way to eat, instead of going on perpetual diets and that we definitely start to make life style changes. The only way to do it now or to do it fast is to start now and start fast .... eating right!

The things to start now and start fast, are drinking lots of water (6 to 8 glasses a day) which washes out the toxins and fat as weight is lost and add daily exercise. Eat lots of fresh fruits and vegetables (5 to 9 servings a day) and take 1 day at a time instead of rushing the process.

The next thing that we can do every day to help us to reach our weight loss goals quicker is to take our time and really chew every bite thoroughly and to deliberately enjoy it - which will help to fill us up quicker and then we will be satisfied with less food.

Also, let us educate ourselves on the basics of nutrition, weight loss and exercise and find the things that work best for our bodies, then perform appropriate exercises for our body at least 3 times a week.

Above all, let us pray for God's help. The Bible says that without God, we can do nothing (John 15:5), but we can do all things through Christ that strengthens us (Philippians 4:13).

7 CHAPTER

RESOLUTIONS

(ARE YOU RESOLUTE?)

It's that time again when large numbers of people - like at no other time of the year - make resolutions to make changes in their eating, exercise, or other routines (or lack thereof) in their lives.

Resolute means marked by determination. Most so-called resolutions have very little determination in them & are forgotten before the end of the 1st month of the year is over. It is said that it takes at least 21 days to form a habit & 63 days for it to be lasting. Most people aren't resolved long enough for their resolution to become a habit.

Today is the day to begin (or resolve) something - not the beginning of the year or the beginning of the week - NOW!!! In order for us to succeed at anything, eating right, exercising, marriage, we need to be resolute, committed, have a made-up mind to reach our goal - no matter what - no matter how long! If we can be stopped or hindered, we will.

Again, our minds have to be made up to do anything worth doing or we will be stopped. When we decide to eat right, there will be many who will bring our favorite cake, candy, treat, chips, or meal. When we decide to exercise, or do anything else worthwhile, there will be things that will come up to hinder or test our commitment to it.

We need to be passionate about reaching our goals & if we are hindered, or tested, let us not be stopped! We can reach our goals by taking one day at a time. If we mess up, we get up & try again. We must be sold out (100% committed) to our goal in order to reach it.

NEVER GIVE UP!!! - though you mess up 7 times - or 70 x 7 times - get back up & try it again! If we give up on a goal we can never reach it!

It will take a complete lifestyle change in order to reach our goals & not slip back into our old habits.

8 CHAPTER

THE DANIEL FAST

Cleanse Your Body with The Daniel Fast

Fasting, by its simplest definition, is to abstain from food. In its broader definition, it can mean to abstain from certain types of food. We should lead a fasted life - - a life that is not caught up with giving our flesh everything that it wants. When we fast - - purposely denying our bodies & bringing them into subjection, we become sharper mentally, physically, & spiritually.

There are all kinds of fasts. There is a complete fast - - no food - - no water. (This should be a very short fast or it could be your last fast, unless you have special instructions from God.) There is a water fast, a juice fast, 40-day fast, 21-day fast, etc. The fast that I'd like to focus on is 'The Daniel Fast'. The Bible, (in Daniel Chapter 1), tells about Daniel & others of the children of Israel who were captives in Babylon. Some of them, who were good-looking, knowledgeable, & quick to understand, were picked & brought to the king's palace to be taught the language & literature of the Chaldeans.

There was an appointed daily provision of the king's delicacies & wine for these young men. Daniel obtained favor & was given the opportunity, for ten days, to prove that the vegetables & water that he & his companions wanted to have, would make them healthier mentally & physically than the ones that ate the king's fare.

After 10 days, they looked so much healthier than the ones, who ate the king's food, that all of the other young men had to eat the way that Daniel & his companions were eating. This has been called 'The Daniel Fast'. Have you ever fasted? When was the last time that you fasted? Fasting can be very cleansing & life-changing - - mentally, physically & spiritually.

Try a 'Daniel Fast' where you eat only fruits & vegetables for 3 days, then 7 days, then 21 days. It will give your system a chance to cleanse & rest itself. Try it! You'll love it! You will find a new way of life. Most importantly, try 'The Life' because Jesus is 'The Way, The Truth & The Life' (John 6:14).

9 CHAPTER

FEMALE WEIGHT-LOSS

Why is it Harder for Females to lose Weight (Fat)?

WHY IT IS HARDER FOR FEMALES TO LOSE WEIGHT (FAT) THAN
FOR MALES & KEYS THAT FEMALES MAY USE TO HELP
THE PROCESS OF WEIGHT (FAT) LOSS *

Researchers have proven that women's fat cells are larger than men's
because female fat cells have more fat-storing enzymes & male fat cells are
smaller because they have more fat-releasing enzymes. Women's fat cells
are twice as efficient in storing fat & enlarging than in releasing fat &
shrinking.

Estrogen is a hormone produced by the female that protects the fat
cells in women & makes it more efficient in storing fat. Female
bodies are made to store fat because the fat is used during pregnancy to
protect & nourish the fetus & for nursing the baby after it's born.

The more a women diets, the more her body tries to protect the fat that
she has & the more the number of fat-storing cells increase & the more the
number of fat-releasing cells decrease. Once fat cells are full to their
capacity, they multiply.

The things that cause female fat cells to produce naturally are puberty & pregnancy. Then there are other things that we do that we can control or stop doing to help our bodies to start to lose weight.

Dieting, overeating, late-night eating, high-fat eating, skipping meals, inactivity, & oral contraceptives are all things that you do, that you have control over, that effect our fat levels .

Females, this might not be what you want to hear, but it is good to know so that some lifestyle changes may be made in order to get out of some of the dieting cycles & circles that you might have found yourself in & make some changes for the better.

The things that you need to do to stop producing fat cells are: make permanent lifestyle changes by doing consistent, regular exercising, stop dieting, eat smaller meals & drink more water than any other drinks. Eating 5 or 6 smaller meals, rather than 3 large meals will help to facilitate weight loss because the smaller meals help to keep the metabolism stoked & make fat-burning easier.

You also need to slow down considerably when you're eating which gives your body a chance to recognize the fact that you're full to keep you from overeating.

Next, you need to stop eating around 7 p.m. or sooner. Lastly, you need to watch the fat content of your food & the types of fat that you're eating.

Knowledge is power, & the more knowledge that we have about our bodies, the more we are able to effect changes for the better for our bodies.

The greatest knowledge that we can obtain is from the greatest book that there ever was or that will ever be, is the knowledge of the Lord Jesus Christ, who will give us the greatest wisdom that we've ever had because He is The Way, The Truth & The Life (John 14:6).

* Most of this information was taken from "Outsmarting the Female Fat Cell" by Debra Waterhouse, M.P.H., R.D.

10 CHAPTER

(SIX EXTRA ARTICLES)

EXERCISE CAN BE FUN!

There are many forms of exercise walking, running, swimming, aerobics, bicycling & I can go on & on. Personally, I teach aerobics & when I made the comment that I enjoy exercising & that it is fun for me - several of my students moaned in disbelief.

The most important thing to do to get started with an exercise program is to find a form of exercise that you can enjoy, because when you have fun with it, it is more likely to be something you will do on a regular basis. It is important to know the reason & purpose for exercising.

God meant for us to use & move our bodies. Due to the changes from the beginning of time to now - in the way that we do things from walking then, to cars & planes now, to the way that we get our food - growing it then, & grocery stores now, the dynamics have changed on every level of life & society.

Our lifestyles have changed, but we still need to move our bodies. Our level of physical fitness effects the other areas of our lives because all areas of our lives are interrelated. The way that we feel about ourselves physically effects the other areas of our lives. The more fit that we are, the better we feel. Regular exercise gives us an edge physically like nothing else can.

Try it for 21 days! You will more than like it! You will love it & feel so much better!

IS YOUR FITNESS SINKING OR SWIMMING?

Sinking Or Swimming (Floating)

Did you know that when you are eating properly & have enough fiber in your diet that your waste will float in the toilet. Are you floating or sinking?

The eating of plenty of fresh raw fruits & vegetables will not only provide life-producing enzymes for health maintenance, but the vitamins, minerals, antioxidants, & fibers for a healthy colon. When you go to the bathroom, it should only be a long trip if you want to steal away for some quiet time away from the family or some moments of peace of mind or reading - not because you need the time to eliminate. Your solid waste elimination process can & should be just as quick as the process of urination, & it should be at least 1 or more times a day.

There are some people who eliminate waste only once or twice a week or even a month. These people need a serious overhaul of their eating habits & /or their colon.

If you are having an elimination problem, try natural sources of help, like prunes, prune juice, psyllium or senna tablets. Psyllium is a natural fiber that can help with the elimination process. Senna provides a gentle stool-softening effect rather than the harsh effect of some laxatives. Natural foods & remedies should always be our first choice of action. You should try your local health food store &/or try a naturopathic doctor for advice on foods & other remedies & make some lifestyle changes vs. quick fixes might help for the short run.

If you keep on doing what you're doing, you will keep on getting what you're getting.

SOFT DRINKS

Is There Anything Good About Soft Drinks?

Soft drinks by definition are non-alcoholic beverages consisting mostly of carbonated water mixed w/sugar or an artificial sweetener plus various natural &/or artificial flavors & colors.

Most soft drinks contain large amounts of sugar & acids that may lead to weight gain &/or dental decay. Soft drinks also have a high phosphorus content that may interfere w/calcium absorption. The average American consumes 40 gallons of soft drinks a year.

Unless the soft drink is caffeine-free, the caffeine may cause problems with adults or behavior & developmental problems in children. A 12 oz. cola containing 50 mg. of caffeine is the equivalent to 4 cups of coffee in a 175 lb. man. Excess caffeine may raise blood pressure & cause irregular heartbeats. Some soft drinks also contain high levels of sodium.

Both the sugar & the caffeine in soft drinks can be addictive &, according to how many you drink per day, you may experience withdrawal symptoms such as headaches, just as if you were hooked on a "drug", if you try to stop drinking them cold-turkey.

Artificially sweetened soft drinks have their own issues because of the harmful effects that each kind may cause. How many people do you know that have lost weight due to drinking diet soft drinks? Studies have shown that the use of artificial sweeteners may even cause weight gain.

Karen Minnis

Some people drink soft drinks instead of water, but for every soft drink that you consume, you need one or more glasses of water to flush out the harmful effects of the acids & sugar (regular or artificial) that you consume. Soft drinks are very hard on your body!

The bottom line about soft drinks, is that they offer little to no nutritional value. Our bodies are the temple of the Holy Spirit & we should do our best to put the best things possible in them to promote life because - Jesus is The Way, The Truth and The Life.
(John 14:6)

HERBAL HOT FLASH RELIEF

Black cohosh is an herb that contains phytoestrogen. It can be used to relieve hot flashes, night sweats, vaginal dryness, incontinence, irritcbility, anxiety, headaches, & depression.

It is recommended that rather than diagnosing yourself, that you consult an alternative practitioner for a diagnosis of particular menopausal symptoms, assess overall health, discuss medical history, & prescribe dosages of herbs.

Personally, around the age of 46, I started to get some show-stopping cramps -- after 32 years of being virtually cramp-free. I tried evening primrose oil & it worked beautifully. Shortly thereafter, I started to get an occasional hot flash & the evening primrose oil worked beautifully once again & I took it daily.

There was a period of time when I failed to replenish my supply & noticed the hot flashes again, but now they were back with a vengeance.

For about a 2-week period, I would be cold in the air-conditioning in my classroom with a jacket on, until a hot flash started. I'd have to come out of my jacket shortly thereafter & then I'd have to put my jacket back on shortly after the hot flash ended.

I went through this several times during a school day. This same scenario continued in the evenings & at night. I would be under the covers until a hot flash started & then I'd take the cover off until shortly after the hot flash was over.

I even came out of my sleep a couple of times with night sweats. I determined to try dong quai or black cohosh & I found black cohosh first. I'm taking evening primrose & black cohosh daily & I am hot flash & night sweat free! Hallelujah!

I thank God for the herbs that He put on earth & for Him giving man the technology to put them in capsule or pill form. He has some awesome things for us all if we just seek after the truth -- Jesus is the Truth -- He is the Way, the Truth & the Life! (John 14:6).

Decreasing High Blood Pressure

Blood pressure. by its simplest definition is a reflection of how hard your heart is pumping. High blood pressure is consistently higher than it should be whether you are relaxed or stressed. Many people have lowered their blood pressure and been able to stop their medications or to considerably lower the amounts of medication by making some lifestyle changes.

Studies have shown that diet, exercise, and other factors can affect blood pressure in positive ways. We will focus on the potential health benefits which can lower blood pressure for those who are interested in improving their health or the health of someone that they love. Things that can be done to lower blood pressure are:

1.) Improved diet - Eating more fruits and vegetables & focusing on certain foods that have proven to lower blood pressure can make a major difference in blood pressure. The list of foods is growing that can help with blooc pressure - celery*, garlic, fatty fish like mackerel (or taking omega-3 fish oils), fruits, vegetables, olive oil, calcium, potassium, and magnesium supplements; or foods rich in those minerals.

*{2 stalks of celery every day for a week caused Minh Le's (62 yrs. old) blood pressure to drop from a high 158/96 to a normal 118/82. Taken from "Food - Your Miracle Medicine" by Jean Carper}

2.) Reduced sodium intake - You should eat no more than 2.5 grams (which is 2,500 mgs) of sodium in a day, especially if you have high blood pressure. The closer to natural that you eat, the less sodium the food contains. A lot of foods contain sodium naturally, and if you've never paid attention to the amounts of sodium in the foods that you eat, you'll be surprised by the amounts of sodium that you're eating in processed foods. It will take paying attention to everything that you put into your mouth, because practically everything that is processed has some sodium in it, even some sweets and boxed cereals.

3.) <u>Stop cigarette smoking</u> - Hypertension is common among cigarette smokers because it causes the heart to work harder and raise blood pressure. Nicotine increases the heart's need for oxygen and the carbon monoxide in the smoke lessens the blood's ability to deliver oxygen.

4.) <u>Increased exercise</u> - 15 to 20 minutes after physical exercise both numbers in the blood pressure reading drop and even more so when a person has high blood pressure.

5.) <u>Reduced sugar intake</u> - Refined sugar contributes to sodium retention which in turn, raises blood pressure.

6.) <u>Reduced alcohol intake</u> - The more you drink, the higher the blood pressure goes.

7.) <u>Increased deep breathing</u> - Some practitioners of Chinese medicine recommend deep breathing. Practice breathing in through the nose and exhaling slowly for 10 seconds, for a few minutes, 4 or 5 times a day which lowers pressure, increases relaxation, and heightens immune defenses.

Over 50% of the diseases & ailments that people are hospitalized for are preventable or can be cured by a change in diet. My people perish for a lack of knowledge (Hos. 4:6a)

ARE YOU TOO SALTY?

Sodium is a mineral that occurs naturally in most foods. Salt is the most common source of sodium.

We only need about 500 mg of sodium a day to maintain good health. We can easily get this amount if we eat only fresh foods & don't add any salt, because most foods have sodium in them naturally. Have you ever heard of someone being deficient of sodium?

The daily recommended amount of sodium is 2,400 mg which is the equivalent of a teaspoon of salt. Most Americans consume about 4,000 to 6,000 mg a day which is far more sodium than needed.

Too much sodium kills over 150,000 people per year and cripples untold others. Excess sodium can cause high blood pressure, ulcers, excess weight, cravings, fears and jitters; also, over consumption of salt can weaken bones, muscles, nerves, and your heart. Are you too salty?

Most of us are not remotely aware of how much sodium that we are ingesting. 75% of the sodium that is added to food is added when it is processed. There is sodium added into foods that we wouldn't expect it to be in, such as, instant oatmeal, most processed breakfast cereals, vegetable juices, & baked goods. It can be unusually high in cold cuts, frozen meals, diet meals, & even some healthy or organic foods.

Karen Minnis

Listed below are the levels of sodium in a serving of some everyday foods in many American diets:

1 hot dog 600-800 mg

1 Cheeseburger 830 mg

1 Sausage Biscuit 1,050 mg

1 Slice of Pizza 290-490 mg

Fries (small order) 200-410 mg

Average Lean Cuisine Meal 480 mg

Healthy Choice Panini 560 mg

1 Cup of canned chicken noodle soup 1,160 mg

Crisp Rice Cereal (1 cup) 210 mg

Honey-nut Cheerios (1 cup) 269 mg

Potato Chips (about 15 chips) 210 mg

Pretzels (about 16 small) 390 mg

Raisin Bran Cereal (1 cup) 362 mg

Ranch Dressing (2 tablespoons) 350 mg

Italian Dressing (2 tablespoons) 430 mg

Strawberries (1 cup) 1 mg

Grapes (1 cup) 3 mg

1 Grapefruit 1 mg

1 Apple 1 mg

Cooked Broccoli (1 cup-no butter) 10 mg

It is a good idea to pay attention to the amounts of sodium in the foods that you are putting into your body. Your body is the temple of the Holy spirit. When you find the right way - walk in it! Jesus is The Way, The Truth, & The Life! (John 14:6)

Karen Minnis

A QUESTIONABLE SUGAR SUBSTITUTE

Aspartame; A Questionable Sugar Substitute

ASPARTAME (aka Nutrasweet or Equal)
A Questionable Sugar Substitute

Do you have any of the following symptoms on a regular basis?: *depression, numbness, muscle spasms, irritability, insomnia, ringing in the ears, headaches, loss of taste, memory loss, dizziness, heart palpitations, diarrhea, anxiety attacks, joint pain, hyperactivity, nausea, vertigo, tachycardia, tinnitus, confusion, or severe*

intolerance for noise. Do you drink diet sodas, use Equal, Nutrasweet, or any other products containing aspartame? These could be the culprit.

Aspartame (otherwise known as Equal, Nutrasweet, or even Spoonful is a thalidomide molecule composed of aspartic acid, phenylalanine & methanol. Methanol, which is a wood alcohol, once ingested, converts into formaldehyde & formic acid. Formic acid is ant sting poison. Formaldehyde, common embalming fluid, is a Class A carcinogen (cancer-causing agent) & a deadly neurotoxin. Neurotoxins and excitotoxins literally stimulate neurons in your body to death, causing brain damage of varying degrees. Aspartic acid has also caused brain lesions in experimental animals.

Dr. Richard Wartman argues that the phenylalanine portion of the sweetener alters levels of neurochemicals, which could cause behavioral changes.

In 1974, the FDA approved aspartame for consumption, but withdrew its approval 4 months later when evidence showed that aspartame caused malignant tumors in rats. Aspartame was re-approved in 1981. Janet Hall, a certified nutritionist, learned that one of the FDA's own toxicologist gave testimony before Congress that aspartame was proven to cause cancer.

She revealed evidence of a cover-up by several high-ranking government officials that some members of the FDA who approved aspartame for public consumption, later went on to lucrative careers in companies involved with the manufacture of this multi-billion dollar chemical.

In 1992, a study of 632 people with serious and/or life-threatening reactions to aspartame revealed that 47% had severe headaches; over 33% had severe dizziness & instability; 20% had epileptic attacks; 25% had extreme depression which was often accompanied by suicidal thoughts; 25% had memory loss & profound confusion; & 25% had decreased vision or actual blindness.

The average American diet contains 17 pounds of aspartame a year. By 1985, (only 4 years after aspartame's approval) the American public had consumed an amount of aspartame equivalent to 1.66 billion pounds of sugar.

After operation Desert Storm, thousands of service men & women returned home with chronic fatigue syndrome & weird toxic symptoms due to diet drinks cooked in the Arabian sun. At 86 degrees, aspartame liberates methanol in the can.

Many weight conscious Americans sip sugarless sodas all day that contain aspartame which cause them to save carbohydrates and supposedly lose weight.

Small amounts of aspartame might be safe, but the cumulative effect of moderate to large quantities consumed in soft drinks and other foods, especially if consumed with a high carb/low protein snack, could produce side effects.

Many in this nation are addicted to artificial sweeteners & the nation as a whole has never been heavier. *How many of you have lost weight due to diet soda?*

ABOUT THE AUTHOR

Karen Minnis is an aerobics instructor certified by *A/R Christian Aerobics* having completed their *Jump Start Program* July 10, 2001

To hear her aerobics routine music CDs go to:

http://www.cdbaby.com/wtlclub6

&

http://www.cdbaby.com/wtlclub4

The Music is performed by *The WTL Club* (The Way, Truth & Life Club. The band is comprised of Karen, her husband and children.) To hear more of their music, go to: http://www.cdbaby.com/all/thewtlclub

Also, Karen Minnis completed the Professional Career Development Institute's *"Professional Fitness and Nutrition Program"* and received her diploma on April 22, 1997 from their *School of Fitness & Nutrition.*

Karen's Health, Nutrition, & Fitness Manual is a composite of various articles Karen has written and her teachings are biblically based from a Christian perspective using a common sense approach to healthy living.

Karen Minnis and her husband Michael were married in 1983; she is the mother of four children, Michael, Christy, Joshua & Melissa; they are all grow-ups. They help out in the gardens, farmer's market and food pantry and so do some of the grand-children.